Bible reflections
for older people

BRF

The Bible Reading Fellowship
15 The Chambers, Vineyard
Abingdon OX14 3FE
brf.org.uk

The Bible Reading Fellowship (BRF) is a Registered Charity (233280)

ISBN 978 0 85746 617 4
All rights reserved

This edition © The Bible Reading Fellowship 2018
Cover image © Thinkstock

Acknowledgements

Scripture quotations taken from The Holy Bible, New International Version (Anglicised edition) copyright © 1979, 1984, 2011 by Biblica. Used by permission of Hodder & Stoughton Publishers, a Hachette UK company. All rights reserved. 'NIV' is a registered trademark of Biblica. UK trademark number 1448790.

Scripture quotations are taken from *The Message*, copyright © 1993, 1994, 1995, 1996, 2000, 2001, 2002 by Eugene H. Peterson. Used by permission of NavPress. All rights reserved. Represented by Tyndale House Publishers, Inc.

Scripture taken from The Passion Translation (TPT)®. Copyright © 2017 by BroadStreet Publishing® Group, LLC. Used by permission. All rights reserved. thePassionTranslation.com

Scripture taken from the New King James Version®. Copyright © 1982 by Thomas Nelson. Used by permission. All rights reserved.

Scripture quotations from the Good News Bible published by The Bible Societies/HarperCollins Publishers Ltd, UK © American Bible Society 1966, 1971, 1976, 1992, used with permission.

Photograph of Paul Canon Harris © Clare Park 2014. Used with permission.

Poem on page 33 © Maggie Jackson. From *Offertory: Poems from a monastery* (Mirfield Publications, 2018). Used with kind permission.

Every effort has been made to trace and contact copyright owners for material used in this resource. We apologise for any inadvertent omissions or errors, and would ask those concerned to contact us so that full acknowledgement can be made in the future.

A catalogue record for this book is available from the British Library

Printed and bound in the UK by Zenith Media NP4 0DQ

Contents

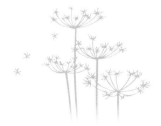

About the writers

Russ Parker was Director of the Acorn Christian Healing Foundation for 18 years before founding 2Restore, a resource for reconciliation and renewal for wounded churches. He is an author and travels extensively as a conference speaker. He is married to Roz and has two children, Emma and Joel. He supports Liverpool Football Club and lives in Surrey.

Sue Richards won *The Upper Room* writing competition in 2017 and this is her first series of reflections for BRF. She lives in Newport Pagnell with her husband and son, and has personal experience of caring for disabled members of her family. She teaches Functional Skills English to adults and has written for a wide variety of magazines and anthologies.

Paul Canon Harris is a poet, writer and broadcaster based in Bournemouth. His published work includes two poetry collections, and non-fiction works on spirituality, leadership and communication. His most recent book is the *Young Person's Quick Guide to Leadership* (Kevin Mayhew, 2018). He is married to Cathy, a speech therapist, and they have four sons, nine grandchildren and a dog called Hope.

'Tricia Williams is a freelance writer and editor with a passion for helping people engage with God's word. She has a special interest in providing spiritual support for people living with dementia and has recently completed research in this area. 'Tricia is married to Emlyn (also a writer for *Bible Reflections for Older People*) and they have two adult children.

From the Editor

Welcome to this new collection of Bible reflections.

If I have a pilgrimage destination, it is Whitby on the North Yorkshire coast. Whitby is what the Celts would call a 'thin place' – a place where the border between spirit and geography is especially permeable. For many years I went on retreat in Whitby, and have twice spent 30 days in silence there, in sight of the ruined abbey on the cliff.

In 2015, in response to the growing interest in pilgrimage, a new route was established: St Hilda's Way. Modest in comparison with some longer, more famous routes, St Hilda's Way wends 40 miles from Saltburn, up over the Moors and back down the Esk Valley to Whitby. One day, I would like to walk St Hilda's Way, but for now my pilgrimage is one of the heart – and as our first writer, Russ Parker, makes clear in his series 'Pilgrim aspirations', this is a perfectly valid form of pilgrimage.

In 2014, the then-Bishop of Oxford, the Rt Revd John Pritchard, inaugurated the Thames Pilgrim Way. This route runs for 104 miles through the heart of the Diocese of Oxford. Bishop John wrote a prayer to mark the opening of the new path. It begins: 'Pilgrim God, you are our origin and our destination. Travel with us, we pray, in every pilgrimage of faith, and every journey of the heart.'

I pray that God will travel with you – and bless you richly – as you journey through these readings and reflections.

God bless you

Using these reflections

Perhaps you have always had a special daily time for reading the Bible and praying. But now, as you grow older, you are finding it more difficult to keep to a regular pattern or find it hard to concentrate. Or maybe you've never done this before. Whatever your situation, these Bible reflections aim to help you take a few moments to read God's word and pray, whenever you have time or feel that would be helpful.

When to read them

You may find it helpful to use these Bible reflections in the morning or last thing at night, or any time during the day. There are 40 daily reflections here, grouped around four themes. Each one includes some verses from the Bible, a reflection to help you in your own thinking about God, and a prayer suggestion. The reflections aren't dated, so it doesn't matter if you don't want to read every day. The Bible verses are printed, but if you'd like to read from your own Bible that's fine too.

How to read them

- **Take time** to quieten yourself, becoming aware of God's presence, asking him to speak to you through the Bible and the reflection.

- **Read** the Bible verses and the reflection:
  - What do you especially like or find helpful in these verses?
  - What might God be saying to you through this reading?
  - Is there something to pray about or thank God for?

- **Pray**. Each reflection includes a prayer suggestion. You might like to pray for yourself or take the opportunity to think about and pray for others.

Pilgrim aspirations

Russ Parker

For the last ten years, I have been leading pilgrimages to Celtic holy sites in the British Isles. For me, the current popularity of pilgrimage reflects a growing restlessness to encounter the presence of God in deeper and fresher ways. Pilgrimage is a reminder that we were not called to a static but to a moving-forward faith. Consider the following quote:

> God's sanctuary is a mobile Ark, his house is a tent, his altar a cairn of rough stones: he leads the Israelites out of Egypt, gives them the solemn feast of Passover and tells them to eat in haste with shodden feet and stick in hand to remind them forever that their viability lies in movement.*

Of course, movement does not necessarily mean moving physically. It can mean moving within: having a constant capacity to grow in God, a constant hunger for more of God, in order to flourish in our circumstances, whatever they are. Even if we find walking difficult or are confined to home, we can still set the compass of our heart to the path of internal pilgrimage.

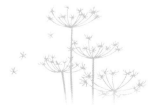

*Quoted by Arthur Paul Boers, *The Way is Made by Walking* (IVP, 2007), p. 39.

Psalm 84:5 (NIV)

A different way to travel

Blessed are those whose strength is in you, whose hearts are set on pilgrimage.

The Message translation has, 'And how blessed all those in whom you live, whose lives become roads you travel.' It evokes the adventure of God exploring our hearts in order to deepen our awareness of his presence in our lives. The whole psalm balances the benefits of being at home in the safety of God's dwelling place with the call to be open to fresh insights and new journeys.

Whether through going on retreat, visiting a holy place or finding spacious quiet in the confines of our home, it is essential that we are always open to discover more of the God who is with us.

Blessing is mentioned three times in this psalm: in verse 4, where it refers to those who know how to be at home with God and keep their worship ever fresh; in verse 5, where it describes the kind of life which draws its strength from God and not itself; and finally in verse 12, which speaks of the one who trusts God with his life. These three blessings sum up what it means to set your heart on pilgrimage.

■ **PRAYER**

Wild Spirit of the living God, be so deeply rooted in me that I know when to be still and when to set my heart on pilgrimage. Amen

Hebrews 12:1–2 (MSG)

Travel light

Do you see what this means – all these pioneers who blazed the way, all these veterans cheering us on? It means we'd better get on with it. Strip down, start running – and never quit! No extra spiritual fat, no parasitic sins. Keep your eyes on Jesus, who both began and finished this race we are in. Study how he did it.

Three essential ingredients for the Christian walk emerge from this text: passion, pace and travelling light. Passion is the business of taking seriously the path we have chosen and fully committing to it. Paul describes the faith journey as a race, but we needn't be intimidated by that idea. If we stay focused on Jesus, he will set a pace we can manage according to our years and abilities.

What we must do, however, is travel light, letting go of anything that weighs us down or holds us back. For Moses, it meant giving up the benefits of a quiet old age as a part-time shepherd. For Paul, it meant giving up his crusade of hate against the new Christians. We may not have the stamina we once had, but the principle of letting go and travelling light in order to press on in our journey of faith applies to pilgrims of all ages.

■ PRAYER
Dear Lord, show me what I need to part with so that I can run the race you set before me. Amen

Psalm 5:3 (TPT)

Travel expectantly

At each and every sunrise you will hear my voice as I prepare my sacrifice of prayer to you. Every morning I lay out the pieces of my life on the altar and wait for your fire to fall upon my heart.

When the French mathematical genius Blaise Pascal died, a piece of paper was discovered sewn into the lining of his coat. It read:

> Year of grace 1654, Monday 23 November, Feast of St Clement… from about half past ten at night to about half an hour after midnight, FIRE. God of Abraham, God of Isaac, God of Jacob, not of philosophers and scholars. Certitude, heartfelt joy, peace. God of Jesus Christ. God of Jesus Christ. My God and your God… Joy, Joy, Joy, tears of joy… Jesus Christ. Jesus Christ. May I never be separated from him.

The psalmist describes his daily practice of making two sacrifices to God: saying his morning prayers and then laying himself, the routine and ordinary detail of his life, before God. Pascal, by contrast, describes a unique, extraordinary moment of intimacy with God when he is spiritually set alight.

Whatever our circumstances, we too can offer the ordinary and everyday to God while keeping our hearts open and expectant for those special times when God brings fresh fire and purpose to our lives.

■ PRAYER

O bright God, help me each day to be expectant for moments of holy fire. Amen

Exodus 33:15–16 (MSG)

Travelling companion

Moses said, 'If your presence doesn't take the lead here, call this trip off right now. How else will it be known that you're with me in this, with me and your people? Are you travelling with us or not? How else will we know that we're special?'

Moses made three epic journeys in his lifetime: the journey to the desert as a fugitive, the journey back to Egypt to demand liberation of his people and the journey to the promised land to create a covenant community for God. But the last journey was disrupted by the episode of the golden calf. Because of the disobedience of the Israelites, God refused to travel on with them and offered Moses a mighty angel as a companion instead (Exodus 33:2).

But Moses wasn't satisfied with this. He wanted – needed – God's presence. Almost any journey is easier if it's shared with someone else, but the core dynamic of pilgrimage is the quest for affirmation that it is God who shares our journey. As we age and lose friends and loved ones, it's God's companionship on the way that becomes ever more important.

We all need the presence of good companions and we can all share in Jesus' promise to his first disciples that he would never leave them nor forsake them: he would always walk beside them.

■ **PRAYER**

Dear Father, wherever my journey takes me, help me know you are with me. Amen

Genesis 28:10–11, 16 (NIV)

Travel with stops

Jacob left Beersheba and set out for Haran. When he reached a certain place, he stopped for the night because the sun had set… When Jacob awoke from his sleep he thought, 'Surely the Lord is in this place, and I was not aware of it.'

Jacob's journey was strewn with his own failures and deceits. He had robbed his brother of his birthright and inheritance and, when his life was in danger, he ran. Yet the place where he stopped became the place of his renewal. Despite his failings, God still had a purpose for his life.

Pilgrimage is a reminder that we all need our stopping places. We visit holy sites not because God is locked up in them but because they challenge us to be open to the God who wants to come closer. Our journey into ageing may bring us to unfamiliar and unwelcome stopping places, but our challenge is to allow them to be places in which God renews our spirits.

■ **PRAYER**

O God of my travels and confinements, guide me to the stopping places where you are waiting to meet and renew me. Amen

Psalm 46:10 (MSG)

Travel with listening ears

'Step out of the traffic! Take a long, loving look at me, your High God, above politics, above everything.' 'Shut up! And listen!'*

This is a psalm of sweeping contrasts. It is a poem about the fact that God favours the city of Jerusalem and lives within its precincts:

> *River fountains splash joy, cooling God's city, this sacred haunt of the Most High. God lives here, the streets are safe.*
> PSALM 46:4–6 (MSG)

The psalmist looks forward to the day when God will end the hostilities ranged against the people of God. Yet, just before the end of the celebration, the reader is commanded to stop and pay attention, lest they miss the true meaning of the words and fail to understand what the writer is saying about God.

In their song 'The Sound of Silence', Simon and Garfunkel sing of people hearing without listening. Listening – really listening – is one of the most important ways we pay attention to God on the journey. It is also one of the best gifts we can give to other people. Dame Cicely Saunders, founder of the first hospice, once said that people will say more in 'a climate of listening'. Real listening is getting harder amidst all the noise and interference of modern life, but if we concentrate hard on giving others the gift of our listening, we can open the way to holy ground.

■ **PRAYER**

Dear Father, help me to listen – really listen – to you; and help me to give others the gift of my listening too. Amen

*Last line: paraphrase by George Verwer, Founder of Operation Mobilization.

Luke 17:11 (MSG)

Travelling the borders

It happened that as he made his way toward Jerusalem, he crossed over the border between Samaria and Galilee.

There are only two references in the New Testament to Jesus entering Samaria. In John 4, he goes to Sychar and asks the Samaritan woman for a cup of water; in today's verse from Luke, he enters a village on the border between Galilee and Samaria. This is where he meets ten lepers crying out for healing, one of whom is a Samaritan.

Jesus walking in this border region symbolises his healing presence in all areas of conflict and prejudice. He challenges us, as Christian pilgrims, to be the people who bring healing and reconciliation in all such places. I remember greeting six Muslim Imams as they arrived at Westminster Abbey to take part in a special reconciliation service on the tenth anniversary of the 9/11 atrocities. I told them that our service would be meaningless without them and thanked them for coming. It opened a whole new chapter of friendship in my life.

■ **PRAYER**
O my God, help me to travel the border lands with you, and do what I can to promote healing and reconciliation. Amen

Matthew 10:42 (NIV)

Travel with little things

'And if anyone gives even a cup of cold water to one of these little ones who is my disciple, truly I tell you, that person will certainly not lose their reward.'

I have led many pilgrimages to the shrine of St David in the cathedral city named after him in south-west Wales. On his deathbed in AD587, he is reported to have said these last words: 'Be joyful, brothers and sisters. Keep your faith, and do the little things that you have seen and heard with me.' A modern equivalent of this was Mother Teresa, who said, 'Do the little things with love.'

God values our every act of kindness and not one of them goes unnoticed, however small. And 'little' does not imply grudging or half-hearted. I am struck by the fact that the verse says 'cold' water, suggesting that effort and attention have gone into this 'little' kindness. Whatever our limitations, if we give such little things the best commitment we can, it says how much we value the other. We are not to serve our fellow pilgrims half-heartedly, but to be creative and fully alive in our caregiving.

■ **PRAYER**

Dear Father God, help me to do the little things well. Amen

Isaiah 40:29–31 (MSG)

Travel and waiting

He energises those who get tired… Even young people tire and drop out, young folk in their prime stumble and fall. But those who wait upon God get fresh strength. They spread their wings and soar like eagles, they run and don't get tired, they walk and don't lag behind.

Most of us are not very good at waiting. We all have our adult version of 'Are we nearly there yet?'. Yet it's surprising how long some of us will wait for the thing that matters. My friend John Presdee visited a synagogue in Bosnia Herzegovina to apologise for the persecution of Jews during the Crusades. He inadvertently left his written statement in his hotel room and asked for ten minutes to fetch it. The Rabbi said that they had been waiting 900 years for this apology; ten more minutes wasn't going to make much difference.

What, then, is a good way to wait? We wait in hope for the Lord for he is our strength and shield (Psalm 33:20). We wait patiently for him and we do not fret when people succeed in their wicked schemes (Psalm 37:7) and we wait eagerly for our adoption as sons and daughters (Romans 8:23). It is this pressing into God that gives us the wings to fly, the energy to run or the power to walk, step by careful step.

■ PRAYER
Dear God, let me know you are there in my waiting. Amen

Exodus 6:4 (NKJV)

Travellers of the heart

I have also established my covenant with them, to give them the land of Canaan, the land of their pilgrimage.

It is not often we get to see the preparations for the birth of a nation. These words spoken to Moses beside the burning bush concerned a disparate group of families that had been in captivity for over 400 years. The founding concept for this new nation was not merely to settle down but to retain a pilgrim heart so that they would continue to be travellers of the heart. Sadly, once established in the land, the nation lost its hunger for God and ultimately this led to the loss of the land itself.

The challenge for all of us, no matter what our limitations, is to be people on a journey of continual discovery about God. Michael Mayne, the former Dean of Westminster Abbey, wrote a wonderful book entitled *This Sunrise of Wonder* (DLT, 2008). In it, he challenges us never to lose the childlike capacity for being open to surprises in the everyday as well as in the exceptional. He wrote this book towards the end of his life while struggling with cancer. He wanted to state that no matter his age or condition, whether housebound or mobile, whether struggling or triumphant, he would not lose his pilgrim heart.

■ **PRAYER**
O God of all long-haul journeys, may I never lose my pilgrim heart. Amen

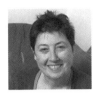

Strength in weakness

Sue Richards

The weakness of God is stronger than man's strength.
1 CORINTHIANS 1:25 (NIV)

I have never been more aware of the truth of those words in 1 Corinthians than one evening some 30 years ago when I was leading the Girl Guide company at church. While we were preparing the hall, I was crushed beneath some heavy room dividers: so heavy, in fact, it normally took six men to move them.

My fellow leaders tell me that they rushed off to find the resident caretaker. When he was nowhere to be found, those four women somehow managed to lift up the room dividers, dreading what they were going to find underneath.

Thankfully, I was still alive, although I'd sustained a tear in my diaphragm, a collapsed lung and a broken pelvis. Later, my other lung collapsed, and I developed a deep vein thrombosis which led to further complications and a two-month stay in hospital. But I firmly believe that it was God who gave my friends their Herculean strength that day.

On the next few pages, we'll look at some of the many ways in which God can use us despite our frailties and make us strong through him.

Psalm 139:15–16 (NIV)

An open book

My frame was not hidden from you when I was made in the secret place, when I was woven together in the depths of the earth. Your eyes saw my unformed body; all the days ordained for me were written in your book before one of them came to be.

Many years ago, soon after we bought our first car, I was facing the prospect of driving down to Swansea from London with my husband, to visit his family. He's been blind since he was four years old, so all the driving responsibilities fell to me and I was frankly terrified. It's one thing pootling around your locality but quite another tackling 200 miles of motorways, country lanes and totally unpronounceable place names.

I was drawn to these much-loved verses in which God gently reminded me that he knew all about my abilities and my nervousness, and therefore I had no need to fear.

Is there something ahead of you that is causing you anxiety? Do you worry that you won't be able to cope with a responsibility that you've been given? If God is calling you to something, however insignificant it may seem, to further his kingdom, won't he also know 'your anxious thoughts' and 'lead you in the way everlasting'? Is it not true, as we've seen already in 1 Corinthians, that 'the weakness of God is stronger than man's strength'?

■ PRAYER

Lord, you know what I have to face today. Take my weaknesses and make me strong in you. Amen

Job 4:3–5 (NIV)

There for others

Think how you have instructed many, how you have strengthened feeble hands. Your words have supported those who stumbled; you have strengthened faltering knees. But now trouble comes to you, and you are discouraged; it strikes you and you are dismayed.

I recently attended the 90th birthday party of a gentleman who has been a fellow volunteer for our local Torch group – an organisation which provides Christian fellowship for people with visual impairment – since it started 25 years ago. He can't do much these days due to decreasing mobility and increasing dementia, but he has a wealth of experience, a great way of explaining things and a very upbeat outlook on life despite some sad incidents in his past. When someone told him that he'd been an inspiration, it brought tears to his eyes, but I really don't think he understands just how much his quiet backstage presence has been appreciated.

It may be his hands that are feeble and his knees that are faltering now but, like Job, he once encouraged youngsters by his patient instruction and served older people with a respectful attitude.

Perhaps now his role is to be that of the 'receiver', enabling younger, stronger souls to serve God as they minister to him. It can be hard to step aside, but someone who enables others to develop their gifts and receives graciously from those keen to be of service is indeed a blessing.

■ **PRAYER**

Heavenly Father, thank you for the opportunities you give us to accept graciously the ministry of others. Amen

Psalm 27:1, 14 (NIV)

He's at work for us

The Lord is my light and my salvation – whom shall I fear? The Lord is the stronghold of my life – of whom shall I be afraid?… Wait for the Lord; be strong and take heart and wait for the Lord.

When my husband and I were in the process of adopting our son from Romania, we were hampered at every turn by bungled bureaucracy, dire phone connections and the fact that it was all such unknown territory, literally and metaphorically. Among many frustrations, one incident sticks in my mind.

Our police checks had gone missing, and with our court date in Romania set for a week away, we needed them urgently. After numerous frantic calls, we were told by someone at police headquarters that the original documents had been shredded and it would take at least two weeks to get replacements.

Just as we were about to despair, the police chief agreed to write us a letter which would be deemed acceptable by the authorities. Apparently, this was completely unprecedented, and it felt like a genuine miracle. I wrote in my diary that night: 'We thanked God for making the seemingly impossible possible.'

If we wait on the Lord and put into his hands those things that seem too big for us to handle, we can take heart and rejoice that he is in control. He doesn't always work miracles, but he does always know what we need.

■ PRAYER
Loving Father, when life seems out of control, help me to hand over to you. Amen

Philippians 4:12–13 (MSG)

Learning to be content

I've learned by now to be quite content whatever my circumstances. I'm just as happy with little as with much, with much as with little. I've found the recipe for being happy whether full or hungry, hands full or hands empty. Whatever I have, wherever I am, I can make it through anything in the One who makes me who I am.

As I use my various prayer guides in my quiet time each morning, I am struck anew by the poverty and persecution, disease and despair that so many of my brothers and sisters in Christ face daily. I don't really know what it means to be in need – compared to them, I have so much – and although I am by no means rich in the eyes of the world, I have plenty of food and enough income to provide shelter, warmth and clothing.

Paul knew what it was like to be in need and to have plenty. He was able to experience peace and contentment in all circumstances – even the harshest – by drawing on God's strength, and he reminds us that we can do the same.

■ PRAYER

Heavenly Lord, give me your strength, so that I too may be content in all circumstances. Amen

Isaiah 41:10, 13 (NIV)

Do not be afraid

So do not fear, for I am with you; do not be dismayed, for I am your God. I will strengthen you and help you; I will uphold you with my righteous right hand… For I am the Lord your God who takes hold of your right hand and says to you, Do not fear; I will help you.

Our son has a number of mental health problems, and I have known times, particularly in the middle of the night, when he has been rampaging around the house, shouting obscenities and punching anything in his way; when I have felt afraid, despite the lock on my bedroom door.

One night, too scared to phone the police in case I was overheard, which would only escalate the situation, I pleaded with the Holy Spirit to fill him with peace and to banish the anger and despair from his heart. I called upon insomniac Facebook friends to summon help, but only one was awake, a friend in Romania, far away and unable to do anything but pray. But as her prayers joined mine, I knew that God had taken hold of me and said, 'Do not fear.' Through the maelstrom of my son's fury, I was no longer afraid.

My son didn't calm down immediately, but God gave me the strength and reassurance I needed to ride out the storm.

■ **PRAYER**
Heavenly Father, when I feel frightened and dismayed, please take hold of my hand and give me strength and peace. Amen

1 Peter 4:12–14 (NIV)

The joy of the Lord

Dear friends, do not be surprised at the fiery ordeal that has come on you to test you, as though something strange were happening to you. But rejoice inasmuch as you participate in the sufferings of Christ, so that you may be overjoyed when his glory is revealed. If you are insulted because of the name of Christ, you are blessed, for the Spirit of glory and of God rests on you.

When we were in the midst of a very troubling situation with our son – facing a court case and dealing with alcohol and drug abuse, as well as health issues and other problems – someone asked me how I could keep my faith. I responded with absolute certainty that I would rather be in that situation with God than not be in it without him. I wasn't happy, but I was joyful because his Spirit was within me.

If we are blessed with the gladness of heart that comes from knowing God, if we are abiding in Christ and daily being filled with his Holy Spirit, then we can rejoice in the limitations and frustrations, the heartaches and sorrows, as well as the good times.

What's more, remaining joyful despite our circumstances can be a very real way to witness to others about our loving Lord.

■ **PRAYER**
Lord, help me to know and to show your joy in my life day by day, that others may see you in me. Amen

Ephesians 3:14–17 (NIV)

It will come from him

For this reason I kneel before the Father, from whom every family in heaven and on earth derives its name. I pray that out of his glorious riches he may strengthen you with power through his Spirit in your inner being, so that Christ may dwell in your hearts through faith.

On our Torch holidays, we always recruit a local speaker and musician and visit an accessible church. One year, we'd found a speaker and a church but not a musician. On the day we left home we still had no one, although we packed the keyboard believing that God would meet our needs. We went to church on Sunday but still no one had volunteered, so I gently reminded the Lord again. Afterwards, a lady came up to me and diffidently offered her services, unsure if she was any good.

She was an extremely competent player and, blind in one eye, sympathetic to our group. What's more, the minister had had no idea she could play. I like to think that, as well as meeting our needs, it was the start of a new ministry for her.

God knew our need for a pianist and also knew what our pianist needed. We had to trust in God's provision and she had to draw on his strength to give her the confidence to offer us her help. It was a match made in heaven.

■ PRAYER

Lord, thank you that you know all our needs: help us always to trust you to help us. Amen

Psalm 119:27–30 (NIV)

Strength beyond sorrow

Cause me to understand the way of your precepts, that I may meditate on your wonderful deeds. My soul is weary with sorrow; strengthen me according to your word. Keep me from deceitful ways; be gracious to me and teach me your law. I have chosen the way of faithfulness; I have set my heart on your laws.

When the mother of our son's daughter walked out of our house, which had been her home for nearly two years, she took our six-month-old granddaughter with her. Despite her promise always to stay in touch, I thought my heart would break.

She broke her promise and, after years of trying to gain access to our granddaughter through the family courts, we gave up the legal fight. We continued to send her presents and cards, but we don't believe she ever received them.

More than ten years later, we still haven't seen her. Even now, our disappointment and despair are hardly bearable at times. Every time our contemporaries become grandparents, the wound is reopened.

I cannot understand God's purpose in this, but I know his word strengthens me and enables me to hold fast to the way that he has set before me. And I know I mustn't let the sorrows in my life hold me back from experiencing the joy that comes from trusting in him.

■ PRAYER

Lord, help me to let go of everything that causes me to stumble and to remember that you have set my heart free. Amen

2 Corinthians 12:9–10 (NIV)

Perfect in weakness

But he said to me, 'My grace is sufficient for you, for my power is made perfect in weakness.' Therefore I will boast all the more gladly about my weaknesses, so that Christ's power may rest on me. That is why, for Christ's sake, I delight in weaknesses, in insults, in hardships, in persecutions, in difficulties. For when I am weak, then I am strong.

A few years ago, my husband and I attended a conference entitled 'Enabling Church', where speakers shared their insights on disability through a biblical perspective and stimulated dialogue about inclusion and involvement in church life. As I've mentioned, my husband is blind. He also has to use a wheelchair. We both led the local Torch group for some years and I helped to run our local Prospects group for adults with learning disabilities, so we were well within our comfort zone at the conference.

As we entered, the worship time had started. It was so heartening and uplifting to see several signers, guide dogs, people reading Braille and others in wheelchairs all worshipping with passion.

In the eyes of the world, many of these people would have been held in little account, but in God's eyes and therefore in ours, those weaknesses merely serve to show his strength and we can be glad that the weaker we might be, then the stronger he will be in us.

■ PRAYER
Lord, thank you for making me weak, so I can show your strength at work in me. Amen

Psalm 71:17–18 (NIV)

Declaring God's power

Since my youth, God, you have taught me, and to this day I declare your marvellous deeds. Even when I am old and grey, do not forsake me, my God, till I declare your power to the next generation, your mighty acts to all who are to come.

A lady from our Torch group is a force to be reckoned with. She is well into her 90s and looks as if a puff of wind would blow her over. She has severe hearing loss, a painful skin complaint and her memory is very poor.

However, she is such a strong Christian and never misses an opportunity to speak of the Lord and to thank him for his goodness. When she says she'll pray for you, you know she means it and if you ask her how she is, she responds as positively as she can without being dishonest.

She spent her adult life as a wife and mother and has experienced a great deal of sadness in her time. She has never had a position of leadership but she shares her love for the Lord wherever she goes and with whoever she meets. I know she'll happily go on proclaiming his name as long as she has the breath to do so.

She reminds me that we all have the responsibility to share what we have learned from, and of, the Lord with those who come after us.

■ **PRAYER**

Heavenly Lord, help me to keep proclaiming your word for as long as I can. Amen

The Gift of Years

 Debbie Thrower founded and leads The Gift of Years programme. She has pioneered the Anna Chaplaincy model, offering spiritual care to older people, and is widely involved in training and advocacy. Visit **thegiftofyears.org.uk** to find out more.

Debbie writes...

Welcome, and I hope you enjoy mining a rich seam of subjects in this edition of Bible reflections. A recent holiday to Lindisfarne set me thinking about pilgrim paths to many far-flung parts of the world. There's great appeal in spending time in wilderness areas, where the intrusions of modern-day living are kept to a minimum. May these reflections be a form of armchair pilgrimage for you, lending a different perspective on our place in the grand scheme of things.

Each of us has 20:20 vision in hindsight. The what ifs and if onlys of the past can disturb our peace of mind if we're not careful. So these reflections are an antidote to negative feelings which might mar the present, if we're prone to dwelling unhelpfully on days gone by.

Oscar Wilde said that his time in jail showed him that 'where there is sorrow there is holy ground... Someday, people will realise what that means. They will know nothing of life until they do.' We're invited to see our times of weakness as fertile opportunities for spiritual growth.

My hope is that, within these pages, you'll find a blend of light and shade. We walk alongside skilful writers sensitively highlighting some of the mysteries of what it is to be human, especially so as years advance.

Best wishes

Meet James Woodward

 James Woodward is the Principal of Sarum College in Salisbury. He is an Anglican priest and has spent the whole of his working life in the Church of England. He was ordained in his early 20s and has been working in a variety of ministries since 1985.

You have a particular interest in the experience of ageing and older people and write and speak widely on this theme. What led to this interest?

I've always felt called to a pastoral ministry; I think people are important and I think making connections is important. I think allowing people to tell their stories – engaging with how people make sense of who they are and what they are – is a fundamental part of the shape of who we are as human beings but also of our distinctive call to living that within the kingdom.

Second, I've always been interested in what theology means in practice and how we put our theological wisdom and tradition to work. So I've been keen to try to understand in a variety of different ways what it means to be faithful to the Christian tradition, and how the Christian tradition might help us to flourish as human beings.

And third, I get very bothered about people and groups with whom I feel we don't engage with enough energy and imagination, and who find themselves on the edges or outside of the care and the love of the community of faith.

So pastoral, theological and a concern for the more vulnerable parts of both ourselves and other people have been the key strands that have brought me to where I am today.

You mention the importance of story. Does the telling of one's story change at different phases of life?

I think we all have a very complicated relationship with our age and there is part of me that would like to have all of the experience of 35 years of ministry and all the security that early middle years brings but still be 30 or 35.

I've asked this question of many, many groups over the past 25 years and I would say that most people have quite a gap between their birth age and how they feel inside. That's reflected a little bit when older people say that one of the most difficult things about being older and hair greying is that people don't see me as an individual anymore. I feel invisible. I feel overlooked.

Some of the theological, pastoral literature says that we go through stages in life and there are tasks associated with each of those stages. I think there are values and beliefs that shape what we think are more important stories or less important stories at different stages. As I grow a bit older, I'm much more interested in synergies and connections and overlaps; I'm much more interested in how telling our stories in the light of our faith experience helps us cope with ambiguity, contradiction and paradox. I think some less healthy forms of religion seek to resolve all those things with certainty and security, whereas our religion at its best helps us to hold our fears and anxieties. We need to find a story with which we can celebrate the limitations: a story that can help us – whatever our age: 35, 45 or 95 – to live with the texture of life at its most paradoxical and ambiguous.

I also want to invite other people in to see what happens when you look at the connections between the dots of our lives, the dots of our story, but to do it within that framework where you value older people, include older people, listen to older people, because that's absolutely fundamental for intergenerational health. We need a community of all ages in order to embrace all ages.

You have a deep concern for 'human flourishing', both personally and academically. What does human flourishing look like, especially in older age?

I think it's about feeling that one's life has been, at least in part, useful and worthwhile, and that the legacy of memory and relationships and work has been recognised as valuable and worthwhile. It's to do with a sense of legacy and being able to think that I may have made a mess of x or y but, on the whole, this has been a life well lived.

It's also about holding one's own human boundedness and vulnerability and limitation and saying to the world outside: 'My value doesn't depend on my mental powers.' There is instead a cherishing of the soul, spirit and heart, of the simple things that matter, of colour and life and movement, and a rejoicing in the world around you. There is the feeling that you've done as much as you can to leave the world a little better, through your children or your grandchildren, or some of the work you've done or, dare I say it, deciding to leave £10 or £20 or £200,000. Our capacity for being able to do good is infinite and some of our flourishing may be found in a capacity for generosity.

The other thing is the feeling that we've been faithful, that we've done our best on our spiritual journey to know how Christ would have us live; that we've prayed for others; that we've continued to hope as society and the church change. When I was ordained in 1985, there were over three million Anglicans in church every Sunday morning and now there are just over a million. We are living in a changing church in a changing world and I think the older generation can teach us how not to give up hope: how to keep the faith.

But if you wanted me to tweet the essence of all that, it's living in the present moment and cherishing the present moment even if that is simply two people together in silence. Words matter less than presence. In the moment, presence is what matters. Learning to cherish this moment is the best we can do. Living in the moment is precious, life-giving and transformative.

An Easter Garden

*I will go to the garden of my heart
and kneel there in the presence of my God.
I will clear winter's leaf-drifts,
with the robin and the blackbird as my help-mates.*

*I will dig black-brown earth into readiness,
and its warmth will cherish seeds to life.
I will plant roses and sweet herbs for His table,
herbs of grace to share with my Lord.*

*I will water my garden with tears of joy.
I will rest from my work in dappled sunlight.
I will sit with my Lord in dappled sunshade,
resting and watching this garden grow.*

*I will watch and wait with the Lord my God,
and in the glory of each paschal morning
He will greet me here and will know my face:
I will meet Him here and will know His grace.*

Maggie Jackson (used with kind permission)

Maggie Jackson is a spiritual director, retreat guide and poet. Having trained in Ignatian spirituality, she has been a retreat guide at the Community of the Resurrection in Mirfield since 2010. She has published poems in several anthologies and on websites, has given public poetry readings and led workshops linking poetry and spirituality. Maggie was Poet in Residence at Mirfield in 2017 and this poem comes from the collection *Offertory* (Mirfield Publication, 2018), which is the published outcome of her residency.

She recalls: 'Some poems emerged from prayer, others from observation or conversation, and prolonged silence stirred memories which demanded to be shared poetically.'

Meet Sue Richards

Sue Richards won BRF's *The Upper Room* writing competition in 2017. She has a background in teaching and social work and currently teaches Functional Skills English to adults. In her spare time, she leads the Milton Keynes Torch Fellowship for visually impaired people. Sue lives in Newport Pagnell with her husband and son. She is a member of the Association of Christian Writers and has had work published in a number of magazines and anthologies. She was brought up in Winchmore Hill, Enfield, a suburb of north London. She says:

It was a very, very happy childhood. I'm the oldest of four girls. We were all very close and still are today. We were a church family, very Anglican. My parents actually helped start the church, so they were very involved from the earliest days. It was on a new estate some 60–70 years ago and they began meeting in a hall. My dad was churchwarden for years and there's even a window dedicated to my grandfather in the church.

What about school?

I went to a church primary school, on to grammar school and then to teacher training college. I hadn't wanted to be a teacher. People always said I'd make a good teacher, so I rebelled against that idea and decided to be a social worker, but I failed two of my A-levels and had to go back to school for a term and retake them. That was ghastly, but in that time I changed tack and decided to be a teacher for special needs children. So I went to King Alfred's College in Winchester to train.

How did your faith develop?

I was confirmed when I was 13 but I remember going to see 'The Cross and the Switchblade' when I was about 18 and this very eager young chap asked me afterwards if I wanted to dedicate my life to God, or words to that effect. I thought 'Oh! Don't think so! That sounds a bit extreme.'

Then I went to college, a year late because of having to do resits, and I happened to find myself in a shared house with two Christians. We all had very similar backgrounds and I decided to join the Christian Union because I thought I was a Christian and I went to a house party run by the Christian Union very soon after I arrived in Winchester. That was when everything changed. I realised that I didn't have a personal relationship with God and I hadn't dedicated my life to Jesus, so I was prayed for there and then. When I came home at the end of the weekend, I prayed with a friend in the house and that's the moment I think I really began as a true Christian. I had the background but my personal commitment wasn't there until that weekend, when I was 19.

How did you go on professionally after college?

There wasn't anything immediately available in Winchester, so I went back home, and just around the corner there was a school for handicapped children – as they were called in those days – but it was for physical handicaps and I was more interested in working with people with learning disabilities. But they needed a teacher and my dad knew the headmaster and he said, 'Oh, my daughter's just come back from college, I'm sure she could help out.' So, I went along for a term and I stayed seven and a half years. I absolutely loved it.

What was at the heart of your love for the work?

It was the learners! Giving the learners the chance to improve and change their lives. But after seven years I moved with my husband – I'd got married while I was there – to Milton Keynes, where I became a rehab officer for adults with learning difficulties. I really enjoyed that because it was a mix of social work and teaching, so it ticked all my boxes.

I stopped being a rehab officer because we adopted our son from Romania and it was such a joy to have him, I didn't want to go back to work until he was thriving. He was 18 months old but he'd been in an orphanage since he was born so he was more like a baby than an 18-month-old toddler. It was a steep learning curve for us all, but there was a lot of joy along the way. By the time he was six, I thought it was time for me to get back into work again and eventually I saw an advert for the adult education teacher job I'm doing now, and have been doing for the last 19–20 years. And, again, I absolutely love the work: it's turning lights on in people's brains and helping them to understand things they never learned as children or never got told in the first place.

When did you begin as a writer?

Probably when I was six – maybe even younger. I've just always loved writing, from my very first story about 'Clara the Cow' which I wrote up as a little book and gave to my mum as a present.

What are you most longing to convey through your writing?

Well, I think my life is great compared to what so many people experience, but there have been difficulties and huge amounts of sadness too. I suppose I want to convey that sense that God has never left me. Some people might look at my life and ask, 'Why are you still a Christian?', but even though life ain't a bed of roses, as they say, there are still so many positives. As I wrote in one of my reflections, I would rather be in these difficulties with God than not in these difficulties without God. I've got experience of certain things that I would like to be able to present to other people through my writing.

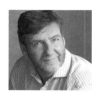

Beautiful hindsight

Paul Canon Harris

Hindsight is a wonderful thing – a phrase usually spoken through gritted teeth with a degree of regret. Christianity is a forward-looking faith with a tradition of remembering – reflecting its Jewish roots. Those who fail to learn from history are condemned to repeating mistakes.

When I was a younger man, I enjoyed rock climbing and hill walking. It was important to fix one's eyes on the summit, the goal – but every now and again, when it felt like a slog, it was wonderful to pause, turn around and see how far one had climbed. It was rewarding and encouraging to enjoy the view in the knowledge that, clouds permitting, even more spectacular sights lay ahead.

Stopping from time to time to review and take stock of the journey thus far is a healthy spiritual discipline. The longer we have been walking, sometimes the harder it is to recall the hopes and excitement we had at the outset of the adventure.

I hope these reflections will remind you of the beauty of hindsight and, if necessary, help you to put any regrets (and most of us have a few) into the more positive perspective of God's great plan.

Exodus 12:25–27a (NIV)

The questions children ask (1)

When you enter the land that the Lord will give you as he promised, observe this ceremony. And when your children ask you 'What does this ceremony mean to you?' then tell them, 'It is the Passover sacrifice to the Lord, who passed over the houses of the Israelites in Egypt and spared our homes.'

Children are naturally inquisitive. They notice things: our habits, our customs and the trinkets we have around us. Their curiosity may cause us to reflect with the benefit of hindsight upon significant events in our past in a way that brings us new insights.

God gave his people the ceremony of the Passover meal as a lasting reminder of his protection and rescue of them in Egypt. He expected that younger generations would be intrigued by it. The expectation was that the older generation would not simply talk about the facts but, rather, that they would say what it meant to them personally.

Younger people involved in my life – family members, friends or carers – may be intrigued by personal customs, the cross that I wear, the prayer book by my bed. From time to time, I expect to be able to explain gently what they mean to me.

■ PRAYER

Lord, thank you for those things that remind me of how you have guided me in life. Help me to share their significance with those who are intrigued by them. Amen

Deuteronomy 5:12, 15 (NIV)

Remember you were slaves in Egypt

Observe the Sabbath day by keeping it holy as the Lord your God has commanded you… Remember that you were slaves in Egypt and that the Lord your God brought you out of there with a mighty hand and an outstretched arm. Therefore, the Lord your God has commanded you to observe the Sabbath day.

'Change is here to stay' is a saying that rings true. Even for those of us who find change a thrill rather than a threat, some changes do feel as if they're not for the best. Sundays are very different from our childhood days; shops open and many people work. My wife's family were very strict about the sabbath – no TV and only games with a Bible theme. As a young girl, she resented some of these restrictions. Now, knowing the busyness of adult life, she sees that they were intended for her good.

God gave the ten commandments for the good of people and society. The Jews had been busy slaves in Egypt, on duty 24/7. Sabbath laws were a gracious gift.

As we get older, the pace of life changes and there can be less variety in our days, yet it is still good to have a special day – a day with a difference.

■ **PRAYER**

God of the sabbath, I pray for people who must work unsocial hours, including Sundays. Please set the pace for my rhythm of life. Amen

Joshua 4:20–23a (NIV)

The questions children ask (2)

And Joshua set up at Gilgal the twelve stones they had taken out of the Jordan. He said to the Israelites, 'In the future when your descendants ask their fathers "What do these stones mean?" tell them, "Israel crossed the Jordan on dry land." For the Lord your God dried up the Jordan before you until you had crossed over.'

Throughout history, people have used stones as reminders about the past, as way-markers, as milestones or, in the case of standing stones like Stonehenge, as places of worship. In Bournemouth, where we live, people leave painted stones hidden all over the place. Children find them and take a photo to post on a Facebook group before re-hiding them. Our grandchildren ask us what they mean.

When the people of Israel miraculously crossed the River Jordan towards the end of their long and tortuous journey to the promised land, they were commanded to take twelve stones from the river bed to pile up at their first campsite. The stones were a reminder to future generations of what God had done.

I was a Boy Scout in my youth and I loved tracking. A small stone on a larger stone was the sign meaning 'gone home'. Scouters sometimes have that on their graves – they have returned home to the promised land.

■ **PRAYER**

Father God, thank you for the milestones and mementoes in my life. Be close to those today who need help finding their way. Amen

Psalm 136:1, 23–26 (NIV)

The one who remembers us

Give thanks to the Lord, for he is good. His love endures for ever…
He remembered us in our low estate His love endures for ever
and freed us from our enemies. His love endures for ever.
He gives food to every creature. His love endures for ever.
Give thanks to the God of heaven. His love endures for ever.

Until now in this series, the focus has been on us exercising hindsight. But the Bible also speaks of God remembering us, which is, when you think about it, a curious expression to use about one who is eternal, over, beyond and around time. Hindsight does not apply to God and that is a beautiful thing.

God may be the Ancient of Days, but he does not have a memory issue, struggling to recall our names or situations. When the psalmist says God remembers us, it means he actively holds us in his thoughts and is constantly and actively aware of us. Perhaps, like me, you have written in a card or email that you are remembering someone in your prayers – meaning you think about them from time to time. God is different – we are always on his radar, objects of his unfailing perpetual love. Thinking about this today may trigger a memory of someone you care about.

■ **PRAYER**
Ageless God, thank you for remembering us who are sometimes forgetful of you. Be close to those I love today. Amen

Isaiah 43:24b–26 (NIV)

He remembers your sins no more

'You have burdened me with your sins and wearied me with your offences. I, even I, am he who blots out your transgressions, for my own sake, and remembers your sins no more. Review the past for me, let us argue the matter together; state the case for your innocence.'

I am the eldest of five children. When I was young, my father went away to theological college. I recall my frazzled mother regularly saying, 'I am tired of your squabbling and fighting.' God, our heavenly Father, uses similar language.

He forgives our sins, blots them out and chooses to 'forget them for his own sake'. It is central to his nature to forgive. This is the amnesia of grace; he actively does not hold our sins and failures against us. It is not passive forgetfulness – it is active forgiveness.

Those of us of the pre-computer era may remember the days of Tippex – bottles of white correction fluid, or later correction tabs slipped in behind the typewriter ribbon. All our mistakes were whitened away like when the Bible speaks of sins being made 'white as snow' (see Isaiah 1:18).

King David implored God 'not to remember the sins' of his youth. Many of us echo that plea. The good news is that God does not remember them. They are dealt with.

■ **PRAYER**

Forgiving God, thank you for your gracious amnesia. Draw close to those who struggle with guilt this day. Amen

Jeremiah 6:16–17 (NIV)

Stand at the crossroads

This is what the Lord says: 'Stand at the crossroads and look; ask for the ancient paths, ask where the good way is, and walk in it, and you will find rest for your souls. But you said, "We will not walk in it." I appointed watchmen over you and said, "Listen to the sound of the trumpet!" But you said, "We will not listen."'

Most of us have watched new bypasses, ring roads and motorways being constructed. I can think of examples where local people campaigned to reduce traffic in their town. Placards such as 'Blanktown is dying for a bypass' were posted on the grass verges. Five years later, after the roads had been built, pleading signs such as 'Turn off now for Blanktown – historic town with attractions and services' appeared as locals fought decline. With the benefit of hindsight, their campaigns might have been different. They may have looked for another solution.

Like God's people through the ages, I have sometimes struggled to find and follow God's way, either through being distracted by novelty or through wilful disobedience. The old well-trodden and proven path of obedience to God is still the best way. Stopping at crossroads and employing deliberate hindsight is necessary from time to time.

■ **PRAYER**
Guiding God, I pray for women and men today whom you have called to be your lookouts and direction-givers. Amen

Luke 22:10–12 (NIV)

A memorable meal

[Jesus] replied, 'As you enter the city, a man carrying a jar of water will meet you. Follow him to the house that he enters, and say to the owner of the house, "The Teacher asks: where is the guest room, where I may eat the Passover with my disciples?" He will show you a large room upstairs, all furnished. Make preparations there.'

There was a pedestrian tunnel near our home which had a great echo. Our boys loved shouting in it. Why do children of all ages love an echo?

The Lord's supper, Communion or however you think of it, is a resounding echo across the years. It is a double echo from Jewish history, celebrating the rescue and deliverance of Passover. It was given a new echo by Jesus' command to his followers to remember him through it: another example of beautiful hindsight.

Among new innovations that I struggle to understand is the 3D printer. Documents from across the world printed out is one thing – toys, weapons and even replacement body parts quite another. The Lord's supper is three-dimensional. We look back, we look around at those with whom we share faith now, and we look ahead to the reunion banquet in heaven: hindsight and future vision gloriously joined.

■ **PRAYER**

Lord, today I pray for fellow Christians throughout the world who are prevented for any reason from sharing the joy of meeting other believers and celebrating the Lord's supper. Amen

Galatians 4:15; 5:7–8 (NIV 1984)

What happened to your joy?

What has happened to your joy? I can testify that, if you could have done so, you would have torn out your eyes and given them to me… You were running a good race. Who cut in on you and kept you from obeying the truth? That kind of persuasion does not come from the one who calls you.

Lend me your ears. Give me your eyes. Paul detects a change of attitude in them towards him, and recognises that it is symptomatic of a deeper, more worrying change. The Christians in Galatia had experienced the freedom that Jesus Christ's grace brings but were lapsing back into legalism. The joy had gone.

Losing your joy is very much like being burgled. You become aware that you have lost something valuable, but you are not quite sure of when and how it happened.

Paul forcefully challenges his friends to stop and look back to see where they had lost their way. At the end of the Bible, the Christians in Ephesus are commended for their perseverance but are also rebuked because they had 'forsaken [their] first love' (Revelation 2:4). As I get older, I want to retain the passion and thrill of the early days of my walking with Jesus.

■ **PRAYER**
Lord Jesus, liberator and giver of joy, I pray today for fellow Christians who struggle to retain joy in the face of life's challenges. Please turn sadness into joy. Amen

Philippians 1:3–6 (NIV)

I thank God every time I remember you

I thank my God every time I remember you. In all my prayers for all of you, I always pray with joy because of your partnership in the gospel from the first day until now, being confident of this, that he who began a good work in you will carry it on to completion until the day of Jesus Christ.

In my schooldays, I was a terror for not finishing my work. I have always been easily distracted – oh look, there's a goldcrest on the bird table in my garden! I am sure I am not the only one whose teachers had to write in red ink, 'Please finish – see me.'

The apostle Paul knew that God always finishes what he starts – no red ink required. Paul's letter to the Philippians is sometimes referred to as the 'Ode to Joy', packed with encouragements to rejoice. He recalls his partnership with them fondly in his prayers, which were ongoing because of memories coupled with looking ahead to a day of completion.

These words remind me that I am a work in progress, one that the author of life will complete in due course. Hindsight enables me to see how God was shaping me even in tough times.

■ **PRAYER**

Loving God, I thank you for joyful memories of people with whom I have shared fellowship in the past. Please keep me open to what you still have in store for me. Amen

1 Peter 3:14–16a (NIV)

Always be ready

But even if you should suffer for what is right, you are blessed. 'Do not fear their threats; do not be frightened.' But in your hearts revere Christ as Lord. Always be prepared to give an answer to everyone who asks you to give the reason for the hope that you have. But do this with gentleness and respect, keeping a clear conscience.

I always think of this as the 'don't jump the lights' verse on faith-sharing. I like to believe I am a safe driver. As an ex-police officer, I should be, but the temptation to jump the lights or to make a quick getaway can be strong. When the amber appears below the red light, you know it is time to get ready.

Peter urged his readers to 'always be prepared' to answer people who seemed interested in or intrigued by their Christian hope. His advice was based on painful personal experience. As a younger man, he had been quick to speak but slow to think. With hindsight, he saw that he had not been ready to answer even a young servant girl who challenged him over his friendship with Jesus (see Luke 22:55–57). Peter's advice in his advancing years was: do not be frightened; be ready; name Jesus.

■ PRAYER

Jesus who restored Peter by the lake, help me to live an intriguing, hope-filled life and to be ready to point people gently to you. Amen

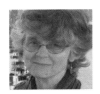

Walking in shadow

'Tricia Williams

Have you ever noticed that sometimes in the darkest, most challenging times, there are surprising moments of joy and lightness? I remember that, when my father died, as well as tears there was affectionate laughter as together my family looked at old photos of his life. I think of friends in terrible situations who recall their sense of God's peace and presence with them in such times. Perhaps you can remember similar examples.

In these reflections, we'll be thinking about some of the shadows of our lives – anxieties, loss, uncertainty. But it's not all bad news. For those who follow Jesus, there is this miracle: in the darkest times, it seems to be there that we find the Saviour and his comfort. Songwriter Stuart Townend has written a song called 'There is a hope'. Indeed there is!

Look out in these Bible passages for words of hope and joy. Whatever shadows you are walking through at the moment, may you know the unseen presence of Christ beside you. May his joy and hope lighten your darkness and give you his peace.

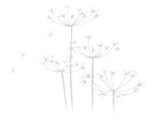

Psalm 23:4 (NIV)

Shadows

Even though I walk through the darkest valley, I will fear no evil, for you are with me; your rod and your staff, they comfort me.

One of C.S. Lewis' Narnia tales is about a 'horse and his boy'. You may have read it. On a long and frightening journey through darkness, the boy becomes aware that there is 'someone' with him, walking alongside, keeping him safe. Later, he discovers it was Aslan, the lion who reminds the reader of God.

Take a moment to think of God's presence with you now. Sometimes in the dark places of our lives, it's easy to forget that God is nearby. We watch the news. We hear of tragedy. We struggle with the heartaches of our family and friends. We feel the sadness of our own frailties or loneliness.

And yet... Here in this shadowy valley of life, we find we are not on our own. Oddly, when we are in the darkest places, it is there we often discover the good Shepherd who walks beside us. Jesus knows all about our human pain and more. It might not make the problems disappear. We may even become aware of the Shepherd's prodding to face up to something, or to move forward. But he is with us. Ultimately, we are safe with him.

■ PRAYER

Lord Jesus, you know about the shadows that I am walking through today. Help me to trust you and to receive your comfort. Amen

Romans 8:28 (NIV)

God has a purpose

And we know that in all things God works for the good of those who love him, who have been called according to his purpose.

I wonder how you imagined your life would turn out when you were a teenager. Do you remember the plans you had? Take a moment to think back over the great things you've achieved, the blessings received, the lives of people you have touched for good. But… do you ever ask yourself in this later stage of life: what is the purpose of it all?

I have several older friends who are facing the challenges of living with dementia. I am humbled and inspired by some who are asking how they can help others in similar tough situations. Here is light in the dark: as Christian believers, we know that even when things go very wrong and are difficult, God still has a good purpose for all his people.

Of course, there's the big plan about how God is bringing people back to himself through Jesus. But there's comfort for each one of us too, in the messy details of our lives, and we can give others comfort as a result. Whatever is happening at the moment, God has your good at heart. And it's not all over yet. He still has plans for you.

■ PRAYER

Lord God, help me be willing today to accept whatever you have planned for me, and to find ways to serve you. Amen

Job 19:25–27 (NIV)

My Redeemer lives!

I know that my redeemer lives, and that in the end he will stand upon the earth. And after my skin has been destroyed, yet in my flesh I will see God; I myself will see him with my own eyes – I, and not another. How my heart yearns within me!

Poor Job. He had lost everything – family, home, belongings, wealth and health. And then, there were his 'friends'. Their words had only brought further torment (Job 19:1–2). It must be his fault in some way. Why didn't he stop complaining? In the midst of his tragedies, Job felt as though he was 'shrouded… in darkness' (Job 19:8).

Then, something miraculous happens. He is suddenly inspired with these words: 'I know that my redeemer lives!' For Job, this assertion of trust in God transforms things. Now, he is sure that whatever his life brings, he will be held safe by God. And his words are prophetic – isn't Jesus the Redeemer, the one who would stand on this earth?

Job's trust points us to Christ, who took our suffering, died and defeated death in his resurrection. We're reminded again that whatever has gone wrong in our lives – our losses, our failures – there's hope and forgiveness in Jesus. Our bodies might be ageing, but with Job we also can assert, 'I will see God!' and yes, sometimes when things are particularly dark and difficult, we probably also 'yearn' for that day.

■ **PRAYER**
Praise God that you are my Redeemer. Amen

Luke 24:1–8 (NIV, abridged)

Surprised by joy

On the first day of the week… the women… went to the tomb… but when they entered, they did not find the body of the Lord Jesus… Suddenly two men in clothes that gleamed like lightning stood beside them… The men said to them, 'Why do you look for the living among the dead? He is not here; he has risen! Remember how he told you…'

Imagine the sadness and confusion the disciples must have felt the day after Jesus' crucifixion. All their hopes and dreams had come crashing down. On that third day, the women came to the tomb to mourn their loss. But there is a big surprise. Jesus is alive. 'Remember what he said?' the angels ask.

Losing a close friend – or a less dramatic loss, like a disappointment, or a failure – may plunge us into all-encompassing gloom. But to us, too, the Holy Spirit whispers, 'Remember Jesus?' Amidst the sadness of our lives, sometimes we're surprised by a gleam of God's light that reminds us Jesus is alive and close by.

These women weren't expecting a miracle. They were just getting on with what good friends and family did in that situation. Into that faithful living, as they were seeking to honour their Lord, God brings his surprising joy. Jesus gives a foretaste of our future resurrection. But even in a troubled present, we might be surprised by God's words of life today. Remember him?

■ PRAYER

Lord Jesus, help me to remember your words of life and joy today. Amen

Romans 5:3–5 (NIV)

There is a hope

Not only so, but we also glory in our sufferings, because we know that suffering produces perseverance; perseverance, character; and character, hope. And hope does not put us to shame, because God's love has been poured out into our hearts through the Holy Spirit, who has been given to us.

It's easy to let our thoughts and conversation be dominated by the things that are going wrong. What is on your heart and mind at the moment? Maybe rejoicing isn't your first response. But the apostle Paul, who wrote these words, encourages us to think differently about suffering.

We know, if we're honest with ourselves, that trials and tribulations are a normal part of everyday life. The early church certainly knew this. So we're not surprised when things aren't easy. The question is, how will we respond? Of course, at one level it is a case of 'keep going': yes, we do need to persevere and keep trusting God, but not out of blind optimism, nor passive acceptance.

Paul describes the link between perseverance and hope. It's important to remember that it doesn't all depend on our efforts. God assures us of his loving presence in the depth of our being through the gift of the Holy Spirit. Whatever our circumstances, our lives can be characterised by his hope – even joy – in the present moment. This hope that God pours into our hearts doesn't disappoint – and may even transform your experience of life today.

■ **PRAYER**

Lord Jesus, may I know the presence of your loving Spirit and the hope that brings. Amen

Isaiah 49:15–16 (GNT, abridged)

God never forgets

Can a woman forget her own baby and not love the child she bore?
Even if a mother should forget her child, I will never forget you…
I have written your name on the palms of my hands.

My memory isn't as good as it used to be. It's not just 'Where did I put my keys?'; I see an old friend and find that, for a moment, I can't remember her name – it's embarrassing. All of us, probably, have such 'senior' moments. For some, sadly, the problems of memory loss are much more significant. But here is good news to store up for shadowy days: God promises that he will never forget you.

Remember the child whose hand you held? Remember the parent who held your hand? This deep bond of loving 'memory' can't easily be broken. We might forget the words which enable us to express our love. We might even fear forgetting God himself. Yet, even if such things were to happen, God will not forget us.

Perhaps you're on your own, you don't have close family and past friends have gone. When you're feeling alone and forgotten, remember this: God has written your name on the palms of his hands – he is always 'mindful' of you (Psalm 8:4, NIV). He never forgets us and he loves us, more than we can imagine.

■ **PRAYER**

Use your hands to help you remember God now. Think of five special memories. Thank God for each of these and his memory of you.

Isaiah 9:2 (NIV)

Light in the darkness

The people walking in darkness have seen a great light; on those living in the land of deep darkness a light has dawned.

Many people around the world are living in places of darkness. Every day on our TV screens and in our newspapers, we see troubled faces, violence and suffering. These words from the Bible were written to the Israelites at a frightening time in their history. They were about to be conquered and taken as prisoners into exile. There would be no easy fixes.

Yet, into this gloom, God speaks his encouragement. The prophet tells of a future when wrongs will be righted, and there will be everlasting peace. These familiar words from our Christmas celebrations remind us of the birth of our Saviour, Jesus: 'To us a child is born… a son is given' (Isaiah 9:6). In Christ, there is God's promise that evil is defeated and Christ the Light will reign forever.

Meanwhile, in this present time, we see glimmers of his light as faithful people risk their lives to bring God's love and healing to others. Perhaps we can't do things like that anymore. But maybe there are ways in which we could share the light of Christ with those around us. How might we bring God's comfort to others today, in the midst of the 'deep darkness' they are experiencing?

■ **PRAYER**
Lord Jesus, be the light in our darkness today. Amen

Romans 8:26–27 (NIV, abridged)

God knows

In the same way, the Spirit helps us in our weakness. We do not know what we ought to pray for, but the Spirit himself intercedes for us through wordless groans… in accordance with the will of God.

'How are you?' a friend asks. 'Fine, thanks,' you reply… and the conversation moves on. Of course, sometimes that's completely true – we are fine. Other times, we might, in fact, be feeling overwhelmingly sad or anxious, and wouldn't know where to begin to explain that to another person. Here's good news for those times.

When we're feeling weak and words fail, we can be sure that God knows our situation. More than that, the apostle Paul tells us in his letter to the Christians in Rome that the Holy Spirit is praying on our behalf. When we don't know what to say, the Spirit is bringing our needs to God, and prays for us in accordance with God's will.

Sometimes, with a very good friend, we don't need to explain how we're feeling. We might even say, 'You know what I mean.' God does know, even better than our best friend, what we mean. He hears our 'groaning' (not grumbling) and the Spirit translates what is on our hearts and brings it before God. Perhaps we can't see how it will work out, but we can trust God's loving plan for us.

■ **PRAYER**

Be quiet before God for a few moments. Thank him that he sees, understands and will answer the unspoken prayers of your heart.

Psalm 63:6–8 (NIV)

In the shadow...

On my bed I remember you; I think of you through the watches of the night. Because you are my help, I sing in the shadow of your wings. I cling to you; your right hand upholds me.

Sleeplessness during the night is a troubling experience. Our worries seem bigger; guilt over things we have or haven't done weigh on our hearts and minds; fears grow with the passing hours; shadows deepen – and we can't rest. David, the psalm writer, knows this experience. Here, he shares some things which have helped him.

When dark thoughts appear, he thinks about God – deliberately and intentionally. Trusting that God wants to help him, he chooses to 'sing' to him. He keeps focused on God, remembering that God is holding him. As Christians, these words 'shadow of...' bring to mind 'the cross'. If our dark thoughts are of past sin, then this shadow can remind us that we are forgiven and put 'right with God' in Christ. We are safe in the shadow of his wings.

When you next find yourself awake in the night time, why not try David's remedies? Meditate on God, sing praise to him. Perhaps pray for others, especially those who are also having a sleepless night.

■ **PRAYER**

'Preserve us, O Lord, while waking, and guard us while sleeping, that awake we may watch with Christ, and asleep we may rest in peace.'* Amen

*From the 'Night Prayer' order of service from the ancient office of Compline.

Psalm 119:105 (NIV)

The next step...

Your word is a lamp for my feet, a light on my path.

Darkness is confusing. We lose sight of the big picture and, unseen, quite small things can seem monstrous. Yet, just a tiny beam of light can change the way we see and feel, and can give us courage to take the next step. In this psalm, God's word is seen as a light in our lives which dispels the shadows.

The psalmist writes in the context of commitment to hearing and living by God's word. Things look different when we start understanding our situation from this perspective. In some ways, it's not difficult. We don't have to know all the solutions, or how it's going to work out in the end. It's just the next faithful step on our path that God's word lights up. And, of course, in that word 'light', we can't help but think of Jesus, the light of the world, who walks beside us holding the 'lamp for my feet'.

I wonder what shadows you are walking through. How might Christ and his word make the next step clearer? Or, maybe you could hold this lamp for someone else who is feeling lost? As we turn to God's word and the one who is the light of the world, may these lighten your path today.

■ PRAYER

'Lead, kindly light… lead thou me on… one step enough for me.'*
Amen

*John Henry Newman (1801–90)

Spiritual care from the cradle to the grave

In 1942, as war raged across Europe and in the Pacific, William Beveridge published a radical report. In it, he argued for a state-run social security system that would fight the 'five giants' – want, disease, squalor, ignorance and idleness.

When World War II ended in 1945, the launch of the Welfare State was announced, and Beveridge's vision became a reality. Among other things, free education, social housing and a national health service (the NHS) providing care 'from the cradle to the grave' would soon be available to all.

The NHS has revolutionised Britain and its commitment to providing lifelong care means that many of us are living longer, healthier lives. Physical and emotional care are important, but they're not the only necessities for true well-being. Research has shown that attending to spiritual needs is just as important for our overall health.

At The Bible Reading Fellowship (BRF), we are passionate about helping people of all ages explore Christianity and grow in faith. Just like Beveridge, we want to provide care from the cradle to the grave. Whether you're a child of five attending Messy Church for the very first time or nearly 95 and enjoying the visits of an Anna Chaplain through BRF's The Gift of Years, we believe we have something that will help you take those important next steps on your spiritual journey.

If you share our vision for transforming lives of all ages through the Christian faith, would you consider leaving a gift in your will to BRF? We value every gift, small or large, and use them for significant projects with lasting impact.

For further information about making a gift to BRF in your will, please visit **brf.org.uk/lastingdifference**, contact Sophie Aldred on **+44 (0)1865 319700** or email **giving@brf.org.uk**.

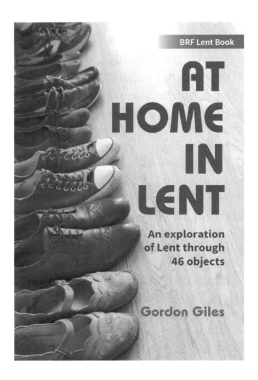

Gordon Giles spends each week throughout Lent in a different room gleaning spiritual lessons from everyday household objects. As a result, you might discover that finding God in the normal pattern of life – even in the mundane – transforms how you approach each day. Running as a thread through it all are the seven Rs of Lent: regret, repentance, resolution, recognition, reconciliation, renewal and resurrection.

At Home in Lent
An exploration of Lent through 46 objects
Gordon Giles
978 0 85746 589 4 £8.99
brfonline.org.uk

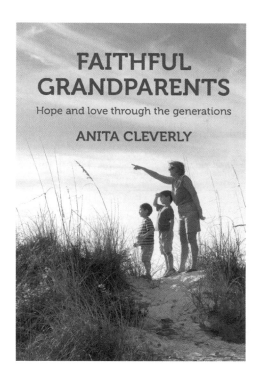

Grandparents can be a vital link between a lived-out gospel and the faith of a younger generation. It takes courage and wisdom, humour and prayer, but the task of passing on the faith appears more significant now than ever before. A visionary book about the privileges and challenges of being a grandparent today; a book which brings soul food to the thriving as well as the hungry, the weary and the disappointed.

Faithful Grandparents
Hope and love through the generations
Anita Cleverly
978 0 85746 661 7 £9.99
brfonline.org.uk

To order

Online: brfonline.org.uk
Telephone: +44 (0)1865 319700
Mon–Fri 9.15–17.30
Post: complete this form and send to the address below

Delivery times within the UK are normally 15 working days. Prices are correct at the time of going to press but may change without prior notice.

Title	Issue*	Price	Qty	Total
At Home in Lent		£8.99		
Faithful Grandparents		£9.99		
Bible Reflections for Older People (single copy)	May/Sep* 19	£5.05		

delete as appropriate

POSTAGE AND PACKING CHARGES			
Order value	UK	Europe	Rest of world
Under £7.00	£2.00	£5.00	£7.00
£7.00–£29.99	£3.00	£9.00	£15.00
£30.00 and over	FREE	£9.00 + 15% of order value	£15.00 + 20% of order value

Total value of books	
Postage and packing	
Total for this order	

Please complete in BLOCK CAPITALS

Title .... First name/initials .... Surname ....

Address ....

.... Postcode ....

Acc. No. .... Telephone ....

Email ....

Method of payment

❑ Cheque (made payable to BRF)   ❑ MasterCard / Visa

Card no. ☐☐☐☐ ☐☐☐☐ ☐☐☐☐ ☐☐☐☐

Valid from ☐☐/☐☐   Expires ☐☐/☐☐   Security code* ☐☐☐
Last 3 digits on the reverse of the card

Signature* .... Date .... /........... /...........
*ESSENTIAL IN ORDER TO PROCESS YOUR ORDER

Please return this form to:
BRF, 15 The Chambers, Vineyard, Abingdon OX14 3FE | enquiries@brf.org.uk
To read our terms and conditions, please visit **brfonline.org.uk/terms**.

The Bible Reading Fellowship (BRF) is a Registered Charity (233280)

BIBLE REFLECTIONS FOR OLDER PEOPLE GROUP SUBSCRIPTION FORM

> All our Bible reading notes can be ordered online
> by visiting **biblereadingnotes.org.uk/subscriptions**

The group subscription rate for *Bible Reflections for Older People* will be £15.15 per person until April 2020.

☐ I would like to take out a group subscription for .... (*quantity*) copies.

☐ Please start my order with the May 2019 / September 2019 / January 2020* issue. I would like to pay annually/receive an invoice with each edition of the notes.* (*delete as appropriate*)

Please do not send any money with your order. Send your order to BRF and we will send you an invoice. The group subscription year is from 1 May to 30 April. If you start subscribing in the middle of a subscription year we will invoice you for the remaining number of issues left in that year.

Name and address of the person organising the group subscription:

Title .... First name/initials .... Surname...

Address ....

.... Postcode ....

Telephone .... Email ....

Church ....

Name of minister..

Name and address of the person paying the invoice if the invoice needs to be sent directly to them:

Title .... First name/initials .... Surname...

Address ....

.... Postcode ....

Telephone .... Email ....

Please return this form to:
BRF, 15 The Chambers, Vineyard, Abingdon OX14 3FE | enquiries@brf.org.uk
To read our terms and conditions, please visit **brfonline.org.uk/terms**.

The Bible Reading Fellowship is a Registered Charity (233280)

BIBLE REFLECTIONS FOR OLDER PEOPLE INDIVIDUAL/GIFT SUBSCRIPTION FORM

To order online, please visit **biblereadingnotes.org.uk/subscriptions**

☐ I would like to take out a subscription (*complete your name and address details only once*)
☐ I would like to give a gift subscription (*please provide both names and addresses*)

Title _____ First name/initials _____ Surname_____

Address _____

_____ Postcode _____

Telephone _____ Email _____

Gift subscription name _____

Gift subscription address _____

_____ Postcode _____

Gift message (*20 words max. or include your own gift card*):

_____

_____

Please send **Bible Reflections for Older People** beginning with the May 2019 / September 2019 /
January 2020* issue (**delete as appropriate*):

(*please tick box*)	UK	Europe	Rest of world
Bible Reflections for Older People	☐ £19.20	☐ £27.00	☐ £31.05

Total enclosed £ _____ (*cheques should be made payable to 'BRF'*)

Please charge my MasterCard / Visa ☐ Debit card ☐ with £ _____

Card no. ☐☐☐☐ ☐☐☐☐ ☐☐☐☐ ☐☐☐☐

Valid from ☐☐☐ Expires ☐☐☐ Security code* ☐☐☐
Last 3 digits on the reverse of the card

Signature* _____ Date _____ /_____ /_____
*ESSENTIAL IN ORDER TO PROCESS YOUR ORDER

Please return this form to:
BRF, 15 The Chambers, Vineyard, Abingdon OX14 3FE | enquiries@brf.org.uk
To read our terms and conditions, please visit brfonline.org.uk/terms.

BROP0119

The Bible Reading Fellowship is a Registered Charity (233280)